Thriving
with
Pancreatic Cancer

*Nutrition, Lifestyle, and Mindset
Strategies for Patients*

Isabella White

Contents

Introduction

This aggressive disease is known for its poor prognosis, with most patients surviving less than a year. When my close buddy Sam was diagnosed with pancreatic cancer, our world and friendship with everyday fun activities turned upside down. The news seemed like a death sentence.

But Sam was determined to beat the odds. He took an active role in his treatment and focused on nutrition, lifestyle changes, and adopting a positive mindset. He became an expert on integrative care and didn't just survive; **he thrived**.

Sam's journey inspired me to write this book. I watched him face the challenges of cancer with remarkable grit and grace. He combined conventional treatment with complementary therapies to heal his body and spirit. Instead of giving in to fear and despair, Sam cultivated an **uplifting mindset.**

In the pages ahead, I'll share the nutrition, lifestyle, and mindset strategies that helped Sam defy expectations. When he was diagnosed, we felt lost and afraid. There was so little information on how to optimize wellness during treatment or improve the prognosis. This book provides the comprehensive guide we wished for.

You'll learn how food can help support your body, evidence-based complementary therapies, stress management techniques, the power of optimism and purpose, and more. Whether you are a patient or caring for a loved one, you'll find tools to boost healing, comfort, and empowerment.

Sam is not only surviving but thriving with pancreatic cancer. This book presents an integrative approach, so you too can defy the odds. By making informed choices, you can take your health and well-being into your own hands. **Be encouraged that there is hope—and actionable steps you can take—on even the darkest days.** Let's get started!

Chapter 1

Understanding Pancreatic Cancer

What is Pancreatic Cancer?

Pancreatic cancer is a type of cancer that affects the pancreas, a small organ located behind the stomach. It occurs when abnormal cells in the pancreas grow and divide uncontrollably, forming a tumor. This tumor can interfere with the normal functioning of the pancreas and can spread to other parts of the body if left untreated.

The pancreas plays a crucial role in the digestive system and the regulation of blood sugar levels. It produces enzymes that help break down food and hormones, such as insulin, that control blood sugar. When pancreatic cancer develops, it can disrupt these vital functions, leading to various symptoms and complications.

Pancreatic cancer is often referred to as a silent disease because it can be challenging to detect in its early stages. The symptoms may not appear until the cancer has advanced, making it more difficult to treat. Common symptoms of pancreatic cancer include abdominal pain, unexplained weight loss, jaundice (yellowing of the skin and eyes), loss of appetite, and digestive problems.

There are different types of pancreatic cancer, with the most common being pancreatic adenocarcinoma. This type of cancer originates in the cells that line the ducts of the pancreas. Other less common types include neuroendocrine tumors, which develop in the hormone-producing cells of the pancreas, and cystic tumors, which form fluid-filled sacs.

Pancreatic cancer is known for its aggressive nature and low survival rates. It is often diagnosed at an advanced stage when treatment options are limited. However, advancements in medical research and treatment approaches have provided hope for improved outcomes and quality of life for patients.

It is important to note that pancreatic cancer can affect anyone, regardless of age or gender.

Causes and Risk Factors

Pancreatic cancer is a complex disease, and its exact causes are not yet fully understood. However, researchers have identified several risk factors that may increase the likelihood of developing pancreatic cancer. It's important to note that having one or more risk factors does not necessarily mean that you will develop the disease, but being aware of these factors can help you make informed decisions about your health.

Age

One of the primary risk factors for pancreatic cancer is age. The disease is more commonly diagnosed in individuals over the age of 45, and the risk increases significantly after the age of 65. While younger individuals can develop pancreatic cancer, it is relatively rare.

Smoking

Smoking is a well-established risk factor for pancreatic cancer. Studies have shown that smokers are two to three times more likely to develop the disease compared to non-smokers. The harmful chemicals in tobacco smoke can damage the DNA in pancreatic cells, leading to the development of cancerous cells.

Family History and Genetics

Having a family history of pancreatic cancer can increase your risk of developing the disease. If you have a first-degree relative, such as a parent or sibling, who has had pancreatic cancer, your risk is higher. Additionally, certain genetic mutations, such as BRCA1 and BRCA2, which are commonly associated with breast and ovarian cancer, have also been linked to an increased risk of pancreatic cancer.

Chronic Pancreatitis

Chronic pancreatitis, a long-term inflammation of the pancreas, is another risk factor for pancreatic cancer. The inflammation can cause damage to the cells in the pancreas, increasing the likelihood of cancerous cell growth. If you have been diagnosed with chronic pancreatitis, it is important to work closely with your healthcare team to manage the condition and monitor for any signs of pancreatic cancer.

Diabetes

There is a strong association between diabetes and pancreatic cancer. People with long-standing diabetes, particularly type 2 diabetes, have an increased risk of developing pancreatic cancer. The exact relationship between the two conditions is not fully understood, but it is believed that insulin resistance and high blood sugar levels may contribute to the development of pancreatic cancer.

Obesity

Obesity is a risk factor for many types of cancer, including pancreatic cancer. Excess body weight, particularly around the waist, can lead to chronic inflammation and hormonal imbalances, which can increase the risk of cancer development. Maintaining a healthy weight through a balanced diet and regular exercise can help reduce the risk of pancreatic cancer.

Diet and Lifestyle Factors

Certain dietary and lifestyle factors have also been associated with an increased risk of pancreatic cancer. A diet high in red and processed meats, as well as a low intake of fruits and vegetables, has been linked to a higher risk. Heavy alcohol consumption, particularly over a long period, can also increase the risk of pancreatic cancer.

Occupational Exposures

Exposure to certain chemicals and substances in the workplace may increase the risk of developing pancreatic cancer. For example, exposure to pesticides, dyes, and certain metals, such as cadmium, has been associated with an increased risk. If you work in an industry where you may be exposed to these substances, it is important to follow safety guidelines and take necessary precautions.

Other Factors

Other factors that may increase the risk of pancreatic cancer include a history of certain gastrointestinal conditions, such as peptic ulcers and gallbladder disease. Additionally, some studies have suggested a possible link between long-term use of certain medications, such as certain types of diabetes medications and statins, and an increased risk of pancreatic cancer. However, more research is needed to fully understand these associations.

It's important to remember that having one or more risk factors does not mean that you will develop pancreatic cancer. Many individuals with no known risk factors still develop the disease, while others with multiple risk factors never develop it. The best approach is to be aware of these risk factors and make lifestyle choices that promote overall health and well-being.

Diagnosis and Staging

When it comes to pancreatic cancer, early diagnosis is crucial for effective treatment and improved outcomes. In this section, we will explore the process of diagnosing pancreatic cancer and the importance of staging in determining the extent of the disease. Understanding the diagnostic procedures and staging system will empower you to make informed decisions about your treatment journey.

Diagnosing Pancreatic Cancer

Diagnosing pancreatic cancer can be challenging due to its location deep within the abdomen. However, several diagnostic tests and procedures can help healthcare professionals accurately identify the presence of pancreatic cancer. If you or a loved one are experiencing symptoms such as unexplained weight loss, abdominal pain, jaundice, or digestive issues, it is important to seek medical attention promptly.

1. Medical History and Physical Examination

The diagnostic process often begins with a thorough medical history and physical examination. Your healthcare provider will ask you about your symptoms, medical history, and any risk factors that may contribute to the development of pancreatic cancer. They will also perform a physical examination to assess your overall health and look for any signs of abnormalities.

2. Imaging Tests

Imaging tests play a crucial role in diagnosing pancreatic cancer. These tests allow healthcare professionals to visualize the pancreas and surrounding structures, helping them identify any abnormalities or tumors. Some common imaging tests used in the diagnosis of pancreatic cancer include:

- **Computed Tomography (CT) Scan:** This non-invasive imaging test uses X-rays and computer technology to create detailed cross-sectional images of the pancreas. CT scans can help identify tumors, determine their size and location, and assess whether the cancer has spread to nearby lymph nodes or other organs.

- **Magnetic Resonance Imaging (MRI):** Similar to a CT scan, an MRI provides detailed images of the pancreas using magnetic fields and radio waves. MRI scans can help evaluate the extent of the tumor and its relationship to nearby blood vessels.

- **Endoscopic Ultrasound (EUS):** This procedure involves inserting a thin, flexible tube with an ultrasound probe into the mouth or rectum to obtain detailed images of the pancreas. EUS can help determine the size and location of tumors, as well as assess the involvement of nearby lymph nodes.

3. Biopsy

A biopsy is often necessary to confirm the presence of pancreatic cancer. During a biopsy, a small sample of tissue is taken from the pancreas and examined under a microscope for the presence of cancer cells. There are different types of biopsies, including:

- **Fine-Needle Aspiration (FNA):** This minimally invasive procedure involves inserting a thin needle into the pancreas to extract a small sample of cells or fluid. FNA can be guided by imaging techniques such as CT or EUS to ensure accurate targeting of the tumor.

- **Surgical Biopsy:** In some cases, a surgical procedure may be required to obtain a tissue sample for biopsy. This may involve removing a portion of the pancreas or performing a laparoscopy to access the pancreas and surrounding tissues.

Staging Pancreatic Cancer

Staging is a crucial step in determining the extent of pancreatic cancer and guiding treatment decisions. The staging system helps classify the cancer based on the size of the tumor, its spread to nearby lymph nodes or organs, and the presence of distant metastasis. The most commonly used staging system for pancreatic cancer is the TNM system, which stands for Tumor, Node, and Metastasis.

Tumor (T) Stage

The T stage describes the size and extent of the primary tumor. It ranges from T0 (no evidence of a primary tumor) to T4 (the tumor has invaded nearby blood vessels or organs). The T stage helps determine the potential for surgical removal of the tumor and the overall prognosis.

Node (N) Stage

The N stage indicates whether the cancer has spread to nearby lymph nodes. It ranges from N0 (no lymph node involvement) to N1 (cancer has spread to nearby lymph nodes). Lymph node involvement can affect treatment decisions and the prognosis.

Metastasis (M) Stage

The M stage indicates whether the cancer has spread to distant organs or tissues. It ranges from M0 (no distant metastasis) to M1 (cancer has spread to distant organs). The presence of distant metastasis often indicates advanced disease and may limit treatment options.

Overall Stage

Combining the T, N, and M stages determines the overall stage of pancreatic cancer. The stages range from stage 0 (carcinoma in situ) to stage IV (advanced cancer with distant metastasis). The stage of pancreatic cancer helps guide treatment decisions and provides an estimate of the prognosis.

It is important to note that staging may also involve additional factors such as tumor grade (how abnormal the cancer cells appear under a microscope) and the patient's overall health. Your healthcare team will use all available information to determine the most appropriate treatment plan tailored to your specific situation.

Understanding the diagnosis and staging process empowers you to actively participate in your treatment decisions. By working closely with your healthcare team, you can ensure that you receive the most appropriate and effective treatment for your pancreatic cancer. Remember, early detection and intervention are key to improving outcomes and thriving with pancreatic cancer.

Available Treatment Options

When it comes to pancreatic cancer, understanding the available treatment options is crucial. Each patient's journey is unique, and the treatment plan should be tailored to their specific needs and circumstances. In this section, we will explore the various treatment options for pancreatic cancer, including surgery, chemotherapy, radiation therapy, targeted therapy, immunotherapy, and clinical trials.

1. Surgery

Surgery is often considered the primary treatment option for pancreatic cancer, especially if the tumor is localized and has not spread to other organs. The goal of surgery is to remove the tumor and any affected surrounding tissues. There are different surgical procedures available, depending on the location and stage of the cancer.

- **Whipple procedure (pancreaticoduodenectomy):** This is the most common surgery for pancreatic cancer. It involves removing the head of the pancreas, the gallbladder, part of the stomach, the duodenum, and the nearby lymph nodes.
- **Distal pancreatectomy:** This surgery involves removing the body and tail of the pancreas, along with the spleen.

- **Total pancreatectomy:** In rare cases, when the cancer has spread throughout the pancreas, a total pancreatectomy may be necessary. This involves removing the entire pancreas, along with the spleen, gallbladder, common bile duct, and part of the small intestine.

2. Chemotherapy

Chemotherapy is a type of systemic treatment that involves the use of drugs to eliminate cancer cells present throughout the body. It can be given before surgery (known as neoadjuvant chemotherapy) to reduce the size of the tumor, after surgery (adjuvant chemotherapy) to destroy any remaining cancer cells, or as the primary treatment for advanced or metastatic pancreatic cancer.

- **Gemcitabine:** This is a commonly used chemotherapy drug for pancreatic cancer. It can be given alone or in combination with other drugs, such as nab-paclitaxel (Abraxane).
- **FOLFIRINOX:** This is a combination chemotherapy regimen that includes four drugs: 5-fluorouracil (5-FU), leucovorin, irinotecan, and oxaliplatin. It is typically used for patients with good overall health and a good performance status.

3. Radiation Therapy

Radiation therapy uses high-energy X-rays or other types of radiation to kill cancer cells or shrink tumors. It can be used before surgery to shrink the tumor, after surgery to kill any remaining cancer cells, or as a palliative treatment to relieve symptoms.

- **External beam radiation therapy:** This is the most common type of radiation therapy for pancreatic cancer. It involves directing radiation from outside the body towards the tumor.
- **Brachytherapy:** In some cases, radioactive material is placed directly into or near the tumor to deliver a higher dose of radiation.

4. Targeted Therapy

Targeted therapy is a type of treatment that specifically targets the cancer cells' unique characteristics, such as genetic mutations or proteins that promote their growth. It can be used in combination with chemotherapy or as a standalone treatment.

- **Erlotinib (Tarceva):** This targeted therapy drug is often used in combination with gemcitabine for advanced pancreatic cancer. It works by blocking the action of a protein called epidermal growth factor receptor (EGFR), which is involved in the growth of cancer cells.

- **Larotrectinib (Vitrakvi):** This targeted therapy drug is used for a small subset of pancreatic cancer patients with a specific genetic alteration called NTRK fusion.

5. Immunotherapy

Immunotherapy is a type of treatment that helps the immune system recognize and attack cancer cells. It can be used in combination with chemotherapy or as a standalone treatment.

- **Pembrolizumab (Keytruda):** This immunotherapy drug is approved for patients with advanced pancreatic cancer whose tumors have specific genetic characteristics, such as high microsatellite instability (MSI-H) or mismatch repair deficiency (dMMR).

6. Clinical Trials

Clinical trials are research studies that test new treatments or combinations of treatments to evaluate their safety and effectiveness. Participating in a clinical trial can provide access to innovative therapies that may not be available otherwise.

It is important to discuss all available treatment options with your healthcare team and consider the potential benefits and risks of each option. Treatment decisions should be made in collaboration with your healthcare team, taking into account your overall health, stage of cancer, and personal preferences.

Remember, every patient's journey is unique, and what works for one person may not work for another. Stay informed, ask questions, and advocate for yourself throughout the treatment process.

Chapter 2

Nutrition for Pancreatic Cancer Patients

The Importance of Nutrition

When it comes to pancreatic cancer, nutrition plays a crucial role in supporting your overall health and well-being. Eating a balanced diet can help you manage symptoms, maintain your strength, and improve your quality of life throughout your treatment journey. In this section, we will explore the importance of nutrition and provide practical tips to help you make informed choices about your diet.

1. **Nourishing your body:** Pancreatic cancer and its treatments can take a toll on your body, making it even more important to provide it with the nourishment it needs. A well-balanced diet can help support your immune system, promote healing, and reduce the risk of complications. By focusing on nutrient-dense foods, you can provide your body

with the essential vitamins, minerals, and antioxidants it needs to thrive.

2. **Maintaining a healthy weight:** Maintaining a healthy weight is crucial for pancreatic cancer patients. Weight loss is a common symptom of the disease, and it can further weaken your body and affect your ability to tolerate treatment. On the other hand, being overweight or obese can increase the risk of complications and hinder your recovery. Therefore, it is important to work with your healthcare team to determine your ideal weight and develop a nutrition plan that supports it.

3. **Managing side effects:** Pancreatic cancer and its treatments can cause a range of side effects that can impact your appetite and ability to eat. Nausea, vomiting, diarrhea, and loss of appetite are common challenges that many patients face. However, with the right nutrition strategies, you can manage these side effects and ensure that your body is getting the nutrients it needs.

4. **Eating a balanced diet:** A balanced diet consists of a variety of foods from different food groups. It is important to include a mix of fruits, vegetables, whole grains, lean proteins, and healthy fats in your

meals. These foods provide a wide range of nutrients that are essential for your body's functioning and healing.

5. **Fruits and vegetables:** Incorporating fruits and vegetables into your diet is crucial, as they are packed with essential vitamins, minerals, and antioxidants that can help boost your immune system and protect you from infections. It is recommended to include a variety of colorful fruits and vegetables in your diet to ensure you are receiving a wide range of nutrients. If you have difficulty consuming solid foods, you can try adding fresh fruit and vegetable smoothies or juices to your diet.

6. **Whole grains:** Incorporating whole grains like brown rice, quinoa, and whole wheat bread into your meals can benefit you in many ways. They contain high amounts of fiber that can help regulate your digestion and prevent constipation. Moreover, they provide a steady release of energy that keeps you feeling full for longer periods. By consuming whole grains, you can maintain a healthy weight and also have the energy you need to cope with the demands of treatment.

7. **Lean proteins:** Protein is essential for repairing and building tissues, especially during cancer treatment. Include lean sources of protein, such as chicken, fish, tofu, and legumes, in your meals to support your body's healing process. If you have difficulty eating solid proteins, consider incorporating protein shakes or smoothies into your diet.

8. **Healthy fats:** It is important to limit saturated and trans fats, but incorporating healthy fats into your diet can be very beneficial. Foods like avocados, nuts, seeds, and olive oil are rich in monounsaturated and polyunsaturated fats, which can help reduce inflammation and support heart health. By including these fats in your meals, you can also improve your absorption of fat-soluble vitamins such as vitamins A, D, E, and K.

9. **Staying hydrated:** It is essential to maintain proper hydration levels for your overall well-being, especially while undergoing cancer treatment. Drinking enough fluids can play a significant role in preventing dehydration, aiding digestion, and eliminating toxins from your body. It is recommended to consume at least eight cups of water every day, and including hydrating foods like

soups, smoothies, and fruits with high water content in your diet can also help keep you hydrated.

10. **Working with a registered dietitian:** Navigating the world of nutrition can be overwhelming, especially when you are dealing with a cancer diagnosis. Working with a registered dietitian who specializes in oncology can provide you with personalized guidance and support. They can help you develop a nutrition plan that meets your specific needs, manage side effects, and address any concerns or questions you may have.

Remember, every person's nutritional needs are unique, and what works for one person may not work for another. It is important to listen to your body, communicate with your healthcare team, and make adjustments to your diet as needed. By prioritizing nutrition and making informed choices, you can support your body's healing process and improve your overall well-being as you navigate life with pancreatic cancer.

Eating Well During Treatment

When you're undergoing treatment for pancreatic cancer, it's crucial to prioritize your nutrition and make sure you're eating well. Proper nutrition can help support your immune system, maintain your strength, and manage side effects from treatment. In this section, we will discuss some strategies to help you eat well during your treatment journey.

Listen to Your Body

During treatment, your body may experience changes in appetite, taste, and digestion. It's important to listen to your body and pay attention to its signals. If you're not feeling hungry, don't force yourself to eat large meals. Instead, try eating smaller, more frequent meals throughout the day. This can help you get the necessary nutrients without overwhelming your digestive system.

Focus on Nutrient-Dense Foods

When you have pancreatic cancer, it's essential to choose foods that are packed with nutrients. Opt for nutrient-dense foods that provide a wide range of vitamins, minerals, and antioxidants. These include fruits, vegetables, whole grains, lean proteins, and healthy fats. Incorporating a variety of colorful fruits and vegetables into your meals can ensure you're getting a good mix of essential nutrients.

Stay Hydrated

Staying hydrated is crucial for your overall health, especially during cancer treatment. Dehydration can worsen side effects and make you feel more fatigued. Aim to drink plenty of fluids throughout the day, including water, herbal teas, and clear broths. If you're experiencing nausea or vomiting, try sipping on fluids slowly or sucking on ice chips to stay hydrated.

Manage Digestive Symptoms

Pancreatic cancer and its treatments can sometimes cause digestive symptoms such as nausea, vomiting, diarrhea, or constipation. These symptoms can make it challenging to maintain a healthy diet. To manage these symptoms, it's important to work closely with your healthcare team. They may recommend medications or dietary modifications to help alleviate these issues. Additionally, eating smaller, more frequent meals and avoiding greasy or spicy foods can also help ease digestive discomfort.

Get Adequate Protein

Protein is an essential nutrient that plays a crucial role in maintaining muscle mass and supporting the healing process. During treatment, it's important to ensure you're getting enough protein in your diet. Good sources of protein include lean meats, poultry, fish, eggs, dairy products, legumes, and tofu. If you're having difficulty meeting your protein needs through food alone, your healthcare team may recommend protein supplements or shakes.

Consider Nutritional Supplements

In some cases, your healthcare team may recommend nutritional supplements to help meet your nutritional needs. These supplements can provide additional calories, protein, vitamins, and minerals. However, it's important to consult with your healthcare team before starting any supplements, as they can interact with certain medications or treatments. They can also help determine the appropriate dosage and type of supplement that would be most beneficial for you.

Manage Weight Changes

During pancreatic cancer treatment, it's common to experience weight changes. Some individuals may lose weight due to a decreased appetite or side effects of treatment, while others may gain weight due to certain medications or hormonal changes. It's important to work with your healthcare team to monitor your weight and make any necessary adjustments to your diet. They can guide you on maintaining a healthy weight and offer strategies to address weight loss or weight gain.

Seek Support from a Registered Dietitian

Navigating the complexities of nutrition during pancreatic cancer treatment can be overwhelming. Seeking support from a registered dietitian who specializes in oncology nutrition can be incredibly beneficial. They can provide personalized guidance, create meal plans tailored to your specific needs, and help you manage any dietary challenges you may encounter. A dietitian can also address any concerns or questions you have about your diet and provide ongoing support throughout your treatment journey.

Stay Positive and Flexible

Lastly, it's important to maintain a positive mindset and be flexible with your eating habits. Some days, you may have more energy and appetite, while other days, you may feel fatigued and have a decreased appetite. It's okay to adapt your eating patterns based on how you're feeling. Remember to be kind to yourself and focus on nourishing your body with foods that you can tolerate and enjoy.

Eating well during pancreatic cancer treatment can be challenging, but it's an essential part of supporting your overall health and well-being. By listening to your body, focusing on nutrient-dense foods, managing digestive symptoms, and seeking support from healthcare professionals, you can optimize your nutrition and enhance your treatment journey.

Managing Digestive Symptoms

Digestive symptoms can be common for individuals with pancreatic cancer, and they can significantly impact your quality of life. These symptoms may include nausea, vomiting, diarrhea, constipation, loss of appetite, and weight loss. Managing these symptoms is crucial to ensuring that you are getting the necessary nutrients and maintaining your overall well-being. In this section, we will explore various strategies to help you effectively manage digestive symptoms and improve your comfort.

Nausea and Vomiting

Nausea and vomiting can be distressing and may lead to a loss of appetite and inadequate nutrition. Here are some tips to help manage these symptoms:

- **Eat small, frequent meals:** Instead of having three large meals, try eating smaller meals throughout the day. This can help prevent your stomach from becoming too full, which can trigger nausea.

- **Avoid strong smells:** Certain odors can trigger nausea. Try to avoid strong-smelling foods or cooking smells that may worsen your symptoms.
- **Stay hydrated:** Sip on clear fluids such as water, herbal tea, or ginger ale throughout the day to stay hydrated. Dehydration can worsen nausea and vomiting.
- **Ginger:** Ginger has been used for centuries to alleviate nausea. You can try ginger tea, ginger candies, or ginger capsules to help reduce these symptoms.
- **Medications:** Talk to your healthcare team about anti-nausea medications that may be suitable for you. These medications can help control nausea and vomiting and improve your appetite.

Diarrhea and Constipation

Pancreatic cancer and its treatments can disrupt the normal functioning of your digestive system, leading to diarrhea or constipation. Here are some strategies to manage these symptoms:

1. Diarrhea:

- **Dietary modifications:** Avoid foods that can worsen diarrhea, such as spicy or greasy foods, caffeine, and alcohol. Instead, opt for bland, low-fiber foods like bananas, rice, applesauce, and toast (BRAT diet).

- **Hydration:** Diarrhea can lead to dehydration, so it's important to drink plenty of fluids. Water, clear broths, and electrolyte-rich drinks like sports drinks can help replenish lost fluids and electrolytes.

- **Probiotics:** Probiotics are beneficial bacteria that can help restore the balance of your gut microbiome. Talk to your healthcare team about whether probiotics may be suitable for you.

- **Medications:** Your healthcare team may prescribe medications to help control diarrhea. These medications can help slow down bowel movements and reduce the frequency of diarrhea.

2. Constipation:

- **Increase fiber intake:** Include fiber-rich foods in your diet, such as whole grains, fruits, vegetables, and legumes. These foods can help promote regular bowel movements.

- **Stay hydrated:** Drinking plenty of fluids can help soften stools and prevent constipation. Aim to drink at least eight glasses of water per day.

- **Physical activity:** Engaging in regular physical activity can help stimulate bowel movements and prevent constipation. Try to incorporate light exercises, such as walking or yoga, into your daily routine.

- **Medications:** If dietary and lifestyle changes are not effective, your healthcare team may recommend over-the-counter or prescription medications to relieve constipation.

Loss of Appetite and Weight Loss

Pancreatic cancer can cause a loss of appetite, leading to unintentional weight loss. It's important to address these symptoms to ensure you are getting adequate nutrition. Here are some strategies to manage loss of appetite and maintain a healthy weight:

- **Eat small, nutrient-dense meals:** Instead of focusing on large meals, try to consume smaller, more frequent meals that are packed with nutrients. Include protein-rich foods like lean meats, poultry, fish, eggs, and dairy products.

- **Try different textures and flavors:** Experiment with different textures and flavors to make your meals more appealing. Adding herbs, spices, and sauces can enhance the taste of your food and stimulate your appetite.

- **Stay hydrated:** Drinking fluids between meals can help prevent you from feeling full and can improve your appetite. Opt for calorie-rich beverages like smoothies or milkshakes if you are struggling to consume enough calories.

- **Nutritional supplements:** If you are unable to meet your nutritional needs through food alone, your healthcare team may recommend nutritional supplements. These supplements can provide additional calories, protein, and essential nutrients.

- **Consult a dietitian:** A registered dietitian can help create a personalized meal plan that addresses your specific nutritional needs and preferences. They can also guide you in managing your symptoms and maintaining a healthy weight.

Remember, it's important to communicate with your healthcare team about any digestive symptoms you are experiencing. They can provide tailored advice and recommend appropriate interventions to help manage these symptoms effectively. By addressing and managing digestive symptoms, you can improve your overall well-being and enhance your ability to thrive with pancreatic cancer.

Supplements and Alternative Therapies

When it comes to managing pancreatic cancer, nutrition and lifestyle play a crucial role. However, some patients may also consider incorporating supplements and alternative therapies into their treatment plans. While these approaches should not replace conventional medical treatments, they can be used as complementary strategies to support overall well-being and enhance the body's ability to fight cancer. In this section, we will explore some commonly used supplements and alternative therapies that pancreatic cancer patients may find beneficial.

Supplements

Supplements are products that contain vitamins, minerals, herbs, or other substances that are intended to supplement the diet. They are available in various forms, including pills, powders, and liquids. While supplements can be helpful in certain situations, it is important to approach them with caution and consult with your healthcare team before starting any new regimen. Here are some supplements that have been studied in the context of pancreatic cancer:

1. **Antioxidants:** Antioxidants are substances that help protect the body's cells from damage caused by free radicals. Some studies have suggested that antioxidants, such as vitamins C and E, may have a protective effect against pancreatic cancer. However, other research has shown conflicting results. It is best to obtain antioxidants from whole foods, such as fruits and vegetables, rather than relying solely on supplements.

2. **Omega-3 Fatty Acids:** Omega-3 fatty acids are a type of healthy fat that can be found in fish, flaxseeds, and walnuts. These fatty acids have been shown to have anti-inflammatory properties and may help reduce the risk of certain cancers, including pancreatic cancer. If you are considering omega-3 supplements, talk to your healthcare team about the appropriate dosage and potential interactions with other medications.

3. **Vitamin D:** Vitamin D is essential for bone health and plays a role in immune function. Some studies have suggested that low levels of vitamin D may be associated with an increased risk of pancreatic

cancer. However, more research is needed to fully understand the relationship between vitamin D and pancreatic cancer. If you are concerned about your vitamin D levels, your healthcare team can perform a blood test to determine if supplementation is necessary.

4. **Probiotics:** Probiotics are live bacteria and yeasts that are beneficial for gut health. They can be found in certain foods, such as yogurt and sauerkraut, as well as in supplement form. While probiotics have been shown to have positive effects on digestive health, their role in pancreatic cancer specifically is not well established. If you are interested in trying probiotics, discuss it with your healthcare team to ensure it is safe for you.

Alternative Therapies

In addition to supplements, some pancreatic cancer patients may explore alternative therapies to complement their conventional treatment. It is important to note that alternative therapies should not be used as a substitute for medical treatment but rather as a way to enhance overall well-being. Here are a few alternative therapies that some patients find helpful:

1. **Acupuncture:** Acupuncture is an ancient Chinese practice that involves inserting thin needles into specific points on the body. It is believed to help restore the flow of energy and promote healing. Some studies have suggested that acupuncture may help manage cancer-related pain, nausea, and fatigue. If you are considering acupuncture, make sure to find a licensed and experienced practitioner who has experience working with cancer patients.

2. **Massage Therapy:** Massage therapy involves the manipulation of soft tissues in the body to promote relaxation and relieve muscle tension. It can be a soothing and comforting experience for pancreatic cancer patients. Massage therapy may help reduce pain and anxiety and improve the overall quality of life. However, it is important to communicate openly with your massage therapist about your condition and any areas of sensitivity or discomfort.

3. **Mind-Body Techniques:** Mind-body techniques, such as meditation, yoga, and tai chi, focus on the connection between the mind and body. These practices can help reduce stress, improve sleep, and enhance overall well-being. Many cancer centers offer classes or workshops on mind-body

techniques specifically tailored for cancer patients. It is important to find an instructor who understands the unique needs and limitations of individuals with pancreatic cancer.

4. **Herbal Remedies:** Herbal remedies have been used for centuries in traditional medicine systems around the world. Some herbs, such as turmeric and green tea, have shown potential anti-cancer properties in laboratory studies. However, it is important to approach herbal remedies with caution, as they can interact with medications and may not be suitable for everyone. Always consult with your healthcare team before incorporating any herbal remedies into your treatment plan.

Remember, while supplements and alternative therapies can be beneficial, they should always be used in conjunction with conventional medical treatments. It is essential to communicate openly with your healthcare team about any supplements or alternative therapies you are considering, as they can provide guidance and ensure their safety and effectiveness in your specific situation.

Chapter 3

Lifestyle Strategies for Thriving

Exercise and Physical Activity

When facing a diagnosis of pancreatic cancer, it's natural to feel overwhelmed and uncertain about what lies ahead. However, incorporating exercise and physical activity into your daily routine can have a significant impact on your overall well-being and quality of life. While it may seem counterintuitive to focus on exercise during such a challenging time, research has shown that staying active can provide numerous benefits for pancreatic cancer patients.

The Importance of Exercise

Exercise is not only beneficial for maintaining physical fitness but also plays a crucial role in managing the side effects of cancer treatment. Regular physical activity can help alleviate symptoms such as fatigue, pain, and depression while also improving your strength, flexibility, and overall endurance. Additionally, exercise has been shown to boost the immune system, reduce the risk of other chronic diseases, and enhance mental well-being.

Types of Exercise

When it comes to exercise, it's important to find activities that you enjoy and that suit your individual needs and abilities. Here are some types of exercise that can be particularly beneficial for pancreatic cancer patients:

1. **Aerobic Exercise:** Engaging in activities that increase your heart rate and breathing, such as walking, swimming, cycling, or dancing, can improve cardiovascular health, increase energy levels, and enhance overall fitness.

2. **Strength Training:** Incorporating resistance exercises, such as lifting weights or using resistance bands, can help maintain muscle mass, improve bone density, and enhance overall strength. It's important to start with light weights and gradually increase the intensity as tolerated.

3. **Flexibility and Stretching:** Stretching exercises, such as yoga or Pilates, can improve flexibility, reduce muscle tension, and promote relaxation. These activities can also help alleviate symptoms of pain and stiffness.

4. **Balance and Coordination:** Practicing exercises that focus on balance and coordination, such as tai chi or gentle martial arts, can help prevent falls and improve stability. These activities can also enhance body awareness and promote a sense of mindfulness.

Getting Started

Before starting any exercise program, it's essential to consult with your healthcare team, including your oncologist and a qualified exercise specialist. They can provide guidance tailored to your specific condition and help you develop a safe and effective exercise plan. Here are some tips to consider when incorporating exercise into your routine:

1. **Start Slowly:** If you haven't been physically active for a while, it's important to start slowly and gradually increase the intensity and duration of your workouts. Listen to your body and take breaks when needed.

2. **Set Realistic Goals:** Set achievable goals that align with your current abilities and energy levels. Remember that even small amounts of exercise can have significant benefits.

3. **Find Support:** Consider joining a support group or finding an exercise buddy who can provide motivation and accountability. Having someone to share your journey with can make the process more enjoyable and rewarding.

4. **Listen to Your Body:** Pay attention to how your body responds to exercise. If you experience pain, dizziness, or shortness of breath, it's important to stop and seek medical advice.

Overcoming Barriers

While incorporating exercise into your routine can be challenging, especially during cancer treatment, there are ways to overcome common barriers. Here are some strategies to help you stay active:

1. **Adapt to Your Energy Levels:** Cancer treatment can cause fluctuations in energy levels. On days when you feel more fatigued, focus on gentle activities such as stretching or short walks. On days when you have more energy, challenge yourself with more vigorous exercises.

2. **Modify Your Routine:** If you experience physical limitations or side effects from treatment, modify your exercise routine accordingly. For example, if

you have neuropathy in your feet, consider swimming or cycling instead of walking or running.

3. **Schedule Exercise:** Treat exercise as an important appointment and schedule it into your day. This will help ensure that you prioritize physical activity and make it a regular part of your routine.

4. **Stay Motivated:** Find activities that you enjoy and that bring you joy. Whether it's dancing to your favorite music, practicing yoga in nature, or taking a scenic walk, incorporating activities that you love will help you stay motivated and committed to your exercise routine.

Remember, every step counts and even small amounts of exercise can make a significant difference in your overall well-being. By incorporating exercise and physical activity into your daily life, you can enhance your physical and mental resilience, improve your quality of life, and thrive with pancreatic cancer.

Managing Pain and Fatigue

Living with pancreatic cancer can bring about various physical challenges, including pain and fatigue. These symptoms can significantly impact your daily life and overall well-being. However, some strategies and techniques can help you effectively manage and alleviate these symptoms, allowing you to maintain a better quality of life throughout your cancer journey.

Understanding Pain

Pain is a common symptom experienced by pancreatic cancer patients. It can be caused by the tumor itself as well as the treatments and procedures involved in managing the disease. It is important to communicate openly with your healthcare team about your pain levels and any changes you experience. They can help determine the cause of your pain and develop a personalized pain management plan.

Working with Your Healthcare Team

Your healthcare team plays a crucial role in managing your pain and fatigue. They have the expertise to assess your symptoms and provide appropriate interventions. It is essential to establish open and honest communication with your healthcare team, as they rely on your feedback to adjust your pain management plan.

Medications for Pain Management

Medications are often prescribed to help manage the pain associated with pancreatic cancer. Your healthcare team may recommend over-the-counter pain relievers, such as acetaminophen or nonsteroidal anti-inflammatory drugs

(NSAIDs), for mild to moderate pain. For more severe pain, they may prescribe opioids or other stronger medications. It is important to follow your healthcare team's instructions regarding medication dosage and frequency.

Complementary Therapies

In addition to medications, there are complementary therapies that can help alleviate pain and fatigue. These therapies can be used alongside conventional treatments and may include:

1. **Acupuncture:** This ancient practice involves the insertion of thin needles into specific points on the body to stimulate healing and relieve pain.
2. **Massage:** Massage therapy can help reduce muscle tension, improve circulation, and promote relaxation, which can alleviate pain and fatigue.
3. **Yoga and Tai Chi**: These mind-body practices incorporate gentle movements, stretching, and breathing exercises, which can help reduce pain, improve flexibility, and increase energy levels.
4. **Meditation:** Practicing mindfulness meditation can help manage pain and fatigue by promoting relaxation and reducing stress.

It is important to discuss these complementary therapies with your healthcare team before incorporating them into your pain management plan. They can provide guidance and ensure that these therapies are safe and appropriate for your specific situation.

Physical Activity and Exercise

Engaging in regular physical activity and exercise can have a positive impact on managing pain and fatigue. While it may seem counterintuitive to be active when you are experiencing these symptoms, gentle exercise can help improve your energy levels and reduce pain. Consult with your healthcare team to determine the appropriate level and type of exercise for you. They may recommend activities such as walking, swimming, or gentle stretching exercises.

Rest and Sleep

Fatigue is a common symptom experienced by pancreatic cancer patients. It is important to prioritize rest and ensure you are getting enough sleep. Establishing a regular sleep routine and creating a comfortable sleep environment can help improve the quality of your sleep. If you are having difficulty sleeping, discuss this with your healthcare team, as they may be able to provide strategies or medications to help you sleep better.

Energy Conservation Techniques

Managing fatigue also involves conserving your energy throughout the day. Here are some strategies to help you conserve energy:

1. **Pacing:** Break tasks into smaller, manageable segments and take breaks in between to avoid overexertion.
2. **Prioritizing:** Focus on the most important tasks and delegate or eliminate non-essential ones.
3. **Planning**: Plan your day to allocate your energy effectively and avoid unnecessary fatigue.
4. **Assistive Devices**: Use assistive devices such as walking aids or reachers to reduce physical strain and conserve energy.

Emotional Support

Managing pain and fatigue can be emotionally challenging. It is important to seek emotional support from loved ones, support groups, or mental health professionals. Talking about your feelings and concerns can help alleviate emotional distress and provide you with coping strategies.

Sleep and Stress Management

Sleep and stress management are crucial aspects of maintaining overall well-being, especially for individuals facing the challenges of pancreatic cancer. Adequate sleep and effective stress management techniques can significantly improve the quality of life and support the body's healing process. In this section, we will explore the importance of sleep, strategies for improving sleep quality, and various stress management techniques that can be beneficial for pancreatic cancer patients.

The Importance of Sleep

Sleep plays a vital role in our physical and mental health. It is during sleep that our bodies repair and regenerate cells, strengthen the immune system, and consolidate memories. For individuals with pancreatic cancer, getting enough restful sleep is particularly important as it can enhance the body's ability to cope with the disease and its treatment.

Unfortunately, many cancer patients experience sleep disturbances due to a variety of factors, including pain, anxiety, medication side effects, and physical discomfort. Lack of sleep can lead to increased fatigue, impaired cognitive function, and a weakened immune system.

Therefore, it is crucial to prioritize sleep and take steps to improve its quality.

Strategies for Improving Sleep Quality

1. **Establish a bedtime routine:** Creating a consistent bedtime routine can signal to your body that it is time to wind down and prepare for sleep. Engage in relaxing activities such as reading a book, taking a warm bath, or practicing gentle stretching exercises. Avoid stimulating activities, such as using electronic devices or watching intense television shows, close to bedtime.

2. **Create a sleep-friendly environment:** Make your bedroom a peaceful and comfortable space that promotes relaxation. Ensure that the room is dark, quiet, and at a comfortable temperature. Consider using earplugs, eye masks, or white noise machines to block out any disturbances that may disrupt your sleep.

3. **Practice good sleep hygiene:** Adopting healthy sleep habits can significantly improve sleep quality. Avoid consuming caffeine or alcohol close to bedtime, as they can interfere with sleep patterns. Limit daytime napping to avoid disrupting your

nighttime sleep. Establish a regular sleep schedule by going to bed and waking up at the same time each day, even on weekends.

4. **Manage pain and discomfort:** Pain and physical discomfort can make it challenging to fall asleep and stay asleep. Speak with your healthcare team about effective pain management strategies, such as medication adjustments or alternative therapies. Using pillows or cushions to support your body in a comfortable position can also help alleviate discomfort.

5. **Seek relaxation techniques:** Incorporating relaxation techniques into your bedtime routine can promote a calm and peaceful state of mind. Deep breathing exercises, progressive muscle relaxation, guided imagery, and meditation are all effective techniques for reducing stress and promoting sleep. Consider exploring different relaxation apps or audio recordings that can guide you through these practices.

Stress Management Techniques

Managing stress is essential for individuals with pancreatic cancer, as it can help reduce anxiety, improve overall well-being, and enhance the body's ability to heal. Here are some stress management techniques that can be beneficial:

1. **Mindfulness and meditation:** Mindfulness involves focusing your attention on the present moment without judgment. Engaging in mindfulness meditation can help reduce stress, improve emotional well-being, and promote a sense of calm. There are various mindfulness apps and guided meditation resources available that can assist you in developing a regular practice.

2. **Exercise and physical activity:** Regular exercise has been shown to reduce stress and improve mood. Engaging in activities such as walking, yoga, or tai chi can help release tension, increase endorphin levels, and promote relaxation. Consult with your healthcare team before starting any exercise program to ensure it is safe and appropriate for your condition.

3. **Support groups and counseling:** Connecting with others who are going through similar experiences can provide emotional support and a sense of belonging. Joining a support group or seeking individual counseling can offer a safe space to express your feelings, share concerns, and learn

coping strategies from others who understand what you are going through.

4. **Time management and prioritization:** Feeling overwhelmed can contribute to increased stress levels. Learning effective time management techniques and setting priorities can help you regain a sense of control and reduce stress. Break tasks into smaller, manageable steps, delegate when possible, and be realistic about what you can accomplish in a given day.

5. **Engage in enjoyable activities:** Make time for activities that bring you joy and relaxation. Engaging in hobbies, spending time in nature, listening to music, or practicing creative arts can help distract from stressors and promote a positive mindset.

Remember, managing sleep and stress is an ongoing process that requires patience and experimentation. What works for one person may not work for another, so it's essential to find the strategies that resonate with you. By prioritizing sleep and implementing stress management techniques, you can enhance your overall well-being and thrive while facing the challenges of pancreatic cancer.

Maintaining a Social Support Network

When facing a diagnosis of pancreatic cancer, it is crucial to have a strong support network in place. The emotional and practical support provided by friends, family, and other individuals can make a significant difference in your journey. In this section, we will explore the importance of maintaining a social support network and provide strategies for building and nurturing these relationships.

The Importance of Social Support

Dealing with pancreatic cancer can be overwhelming, both physically and emotionally. Having a support network can help alleviate some of the burden and provide a sense of comfort and understanding. Here are a few reasons why maintaining a social support network is essential:

1. **Emotional Support:** Friends and family can offer a listening ear, empathy, and encouragement during difficult times. They can provide a safe space for you to express your fears, frustrations, and emotions without judgment.

2. **Practical Support:** Your support network can assist with daily tasks, such as cooking, cleaning, and running errands, allowing you to focus on your treatment and recovery. They can also accompany

you to medical appointments and help you navigate the healthcare system.

3. **Information and Resources:** Your loved ones can help you gather information about treatment options, clinical trials, and support groups. They can also connect you with other individuals who have faced similar challenges, providing valuable insights and advice.

4. **Motivation and Inspiration:** Surrounding yourself with positive and supportive individuals can boost your morale and motivation. Their encouragement and belief in your ability to overcome obstacles can be a powerful source of strength.

Building and Nurturing Your Support Network

Creating and maintaining a social support network requires effort and open communication. Here are some strategies to help you build and nurture these relationships:

1. **Communicate Your Needs:** Be open and honest with your loved ones about your needs and how they can support you. Clearly express what you are comfortable with and what you may need assistance with. Effective communication is key to ensuring

that your support network understands how best to help you.

2. **Seek Support Groups:** Joining a support group specifically for pancreatic cancer patients can provide a unique sense of understanding and camaraderie. These groups offer a safe space to share experiences, exchange information, and receive emotional support from individuals who are going through similar challenges.

3. **Lean on Friends and Family:** Reach out to your close friends and family members and let them know how they can support you. Whether it's through regular check-ins, accompanying you to appointments, or simply spending quality time together, their presence can make a significant difference in your well-being.

4. **Connect Virtually:** In today's digital age, it is easier than ever to connect with others virtually. Utilize social media platforms, online forums, and video calls to stay connected with friends, family, and support groups, especially if distance or mobility is a challenge.

5. **Consider Professional Support:** In addition to your support network, consider seeking professional

help from therapists, counselors, or social workers who specialize in supporting individuals with cancer. They can provide guidance, coping strategies, and a safe space to process your emotions.

6. **Give and Receive:** Remember that relationships are a two-way street. While it is important to receive support, also offer your support to others when you can. Being there for others can provide a sense of purpose and fulfillment, and it strengthens the bonds within your support network.

7. **Explore Online Communities:** The internet offers a wealth of resources and online communities for individuals facing pancreatic cancer. These communities can provide a platform for sharing experiences, asking questions, and finding support from people around the world who understand what you are going through.

Overcoming Challenges in Maintaining a Support Network

While building and maintaining a social support network is crucial, it is important to acknowledge that there may be challenges along the way. Here are a few common obstacles and strategies to overcome them:

1. **Fear of Burdening Others:** It is common to feel hesitant about asking for help or sharing your struggles with others. Remember that your loved ones want to support you, and allowing them to do so can strengthen your relationship.

2. **Changes in Relationships:** A cancer diagnosis can sometimes strain relationships, as people may struggle to understand or cope with the situation. Open and honest communication can help address any misunderstandings or conflicts that may arise.

3. **Dealing with Isolation:** Pancreatic cancer can sometimes lead to feelings of isolation, especially if you are unable to participate in activities or social events as you used to. Stay connected with your support network through phone calls, video chats, or even written correspondence to combat feelings of loneliness.

4. **Seeking Professional Help:** If you find it challenging to build or maintain a support network, consider reaching out to a healthcare professional who can provide guidance and connect you with additional resources.

Remember, you are not alone in your journey. Building and nurturing a social support network can provide you with the emotional and practical support you need to thrive with pancreatic cancer. Reach out to your loved ones, join support groups, and explore online communities to connect with others who understand and can offer support and encouragement.

Chapter 4

Mindset and Emotional Well-being

Coping with the Diagnosis

Receiving a diagnosis of pancreatic cancer can be overwhelming and emotionally challenging. It is natural to experience a range of emotions, including fear, sadness, anger, and confusion. Coping with the diagnosis is an essential part of your journey towards thriving with pancreatic cancer. In this section, we will explore various strategies to help you navigate through this difficult time and find strength and resilience.

Acknowledge Your Emotions

The first step in coping with the diagnosis is to acknowledge and accept your emotions. It is normal to feel a wide range of emotions, and it is important to permit yourself to experience them. Allow yourself to grieve, be angry, or feel scared. Remember that these emotions are valid and part of the healing process.

Seek Support

You don't have to face this journey alone. Reach out to your support system, including family, friends, and healthcare professionals. Share your feelings and concerns with them. They can provide comfort, understanding, and practical assistance. Consider joining a support group for individuals with pancreatic cancer. Connecting with others who are going through a similar experience can be incredibly helpful and provide a sense of belonging.

Educate Yourself

Knowledge is power, and understanding your diagnosis can help alleviate some of the anxiety and uncertainty. Take the time to learn about pancreatic cancer, its treatment options, and its potential side effects. Ask your healthcare team questions and seek reliable sources of information. However, be cautious about overwhelming yourself with too much information. Find a balance that allows you to stay informed without becoming overwhelmed.

Communicate with Your Healthcare Team

Open and honest communication with your healthcare team is crucial. They are there to support you and provide guidance throughout your treatment journey. Don't hesitate to ask questions, express your concerns, or seek clarification about your diagnosis and treatment plan. Remember that you are an active participant in your healthcare, and your voice matters.

Practice Self-Care

Taking care of yourself physically, emotionally, and mentally is essential during this challenging time. Prioritize self-care activities that bring you joy and relaxation. Engage in activities such as gentle exercise, meditation, deep breathing exercises, or journaling. Find what works best for you and make it a regular part of your routine.

Embrace a Positive Mindset

Maintaining a positive mindset can be a powerful tool in coping with the diagnosis. While it is natural to have moments of negativity, try to focus on the things that bring you joy and gratitude. Surround yourself with positive influences, whether it be uplifting books, inspiring podcasts, or supportive friends. Practice positive affirmations and visualization techniques to help shift your mindset towards hope and resilience.

Seek Professional Help

If you find that your emotions are becoming overwhelming or interfering with your daily life, consider seeking professional help. A therapist or counselor experienced in working with cancer patients can provide valuable support and guidance. They can help you navigate through the emotional challenges and develop coping strategies tailored to your needs.

Embrace Spirituality

For many individuals, spirituality can provide solace and a sense of purpose during difficult times. Explore your spiritual beliefs and practices, whether it be through prayer, meditation, or connecting with a religious community. Engaging in spiritual activities can help you find inner peace and strength.

Embrace the Present Moment

Living with a cancer diagnosis can make it easy to get caught up in worries about the future. However, embracing the present moment can help reduce anxiety and bring a sense of calm. Practice mindfulness by focusing on the here and now. Engage in activities that bring you joy, and allow yourself to fully experience them.

Find Meaning and Purpose

Finding meaning and purpose in your life can be a powerful way to cope with the diagnosis. Reflect on what truly matters to you and what brings you a sense of fulfillment. This may involve spending quality time with loved ones, pursuing hobbies or interests, or giving back to your community. By focusing on what gives your life meaning, you can find strength and motivation to navigate through the challenges of pancreatic cancer.

Remember, coping with the diagnosis is a personal journey, and everyone's experience is unique. Be patient with yourself and allow yourself to feel and process your emotions. Surround yourself with a supportive network, take care of yourself, and embrace a positive mindset. By implementing these strategies, you can find the strength and resilience to thrive with pancreatic cancer.

Positive Thinking and Visualization

When facing a diagnosis of pancreatic cancer, it's natural to experience a range of emotions, including fear, sadness, and uncertainty. However, maintaining a positive mindset can have a profound impact on your overall well-being and quality of life. Positive thinking and visualization techniques can help you navigate the challenges of pancreatic cancer with resilience and hope.

The Power of Positive Thinking

Positive thinking involves consciously choosing to focus on the positive aspects of your life and situation rather than dwelling on the negative. It doesn't mean ignoring the reality of your diagnosis or denying your emotions. Instead, it's about shifting your perspective and finding ways to cultivate optimism and hope.

Research has shown that positive thinking can have numerous benefits for cancer patients. It can improve your mental and emotional well-being, reduce stress levels, enhance your immune system, and even contribute to better treatment outcomes. By adopting a positive mindset, you can empower yourself to face the challenges of pancreatic cancer with strength and resilience.

Cultivating Positive Thinking

Cultivating a positive mindset takes practice and intention. Here are some strategies to help you foster positive thinking:

1. **Practice gratitude:** Take a few moments each day to reflect on the things you are grateful for. This can be as simple as appreciating a beautiful sunset, the support of loved ones, or the kindness of a stranger. By focusing on the positive aspects of your life, you can shift your perspective and cultivate a sense of gratitude.

2. **Surround yourself with positivity:** Surround yourself with people who uplift and inspire you. Seek out support groups, online communities, or counseling services where you can connect with others who are going through similar experiences. Sharing your journey with others who understand can provide a sense of camaraderie and positivity.

3. **Practice positive self-talk:** Pay attention to your inner dialogue and challenge negative thoughts. Replace self-critical or pessimistic thoughts with positive affirmations. Remind yourself of your strengths, resilience, and the progress you have made. By reframing your thoughts, you can cultivate a more positive and empowering mindset.

4. **Engage in activities that bring you joy:** Find activities that bring you joy and make time for them regularly. Whether it's spending time in nature, pursuing a hobby, listening to music, or practicing mindfulness, engaging in activities that bring you happiness can boost your mood and overall well-being.

The Power of Visualization

Visualization is a powerful technique that involves using your imagination to create mental images of positive outcomes and experiences. By visualizing yourself as healthy, strong, and thriving, you can tap into the power of your mind to support your healing journey.

Visualization can help reduce anxiety, improve mood, and enhance your overall well-being. It can also help you develop a sense of control and agency over your health, which is particularly important when facing a challenging diagnosis like pancreatic cancer.

Practicing Visualization

To practice visualization, find a quiet and comfortable space where you won't be disturbed. Close your eyes and take a few deep breaths to relax your body and mind. Then, imagine yourself in a peaceful and healing environment. It could be a serene beach, a lush forest, or any place that brings you a sense of calm and tranquility.

Once you have created this mental image, visualize yourself as healthy and vibrant. See yourself engaging in activities that bring you joy and fulfillment. Imagine your body healing and your immune system becoming stronger. Allow yourself to feel the emotions associated with this visualization, such as joy, gratitude, and hope.

You can also use guided visualization recordings or apps to support your practice. These resources provide step-by-step instructions and imagery to guide you through the visualization process.

Integrating Positive Thinking and Visualization into Your Daily Life

Incorporating positive thinking and visualization into your daily routine can have a profound impact on your mindset and overall well-being. Here are some tips to help you integrate these practices into your life:

1. **Create a daily ritual:** Set aside a specific time each day to practice positive thinking and visualization. It could be in the morning, before bed, or during a quiet moment in the middle of the day. Consistency is key to reaping the benefits of these practices.

2. **Use visual cues:** Place visual reminders of positivity and hope in your environment. It could be a vision board with images that inspire you, uplifting quotes, or photographs of loved ones. These visual cues can serve as reminders to maintain a positive mindset throughout the day.

3. **Combine positive thinking with other activities:** Incorporate positive thinking and visualization into

other activities you already do. For example, while receiving treatment, visualize the medication or therapy targeting and destroying cancer cells. During exercise, imagine your body becoming stronger and more resilient. By combining these practices with daily activities, you can reinforce positive thinking and visualization.

Remember, positive thinking and visualization are tools to support your overall well-being and mindset. They are not a substitute for medical treatment or professional support. It's important to work closely with your healthcare team and seek emotional support when needed.

By embracing positive thinking and visualization, you can cultivate a mindset of resilience, hope, and empowerment as you navigate your journey with pancreatic cancer.

Finding Meaning and Purpose

When faced with a diagnosis of pancreatic cancer, it is natural to question the meaning and purpose of life. This journey can be overwhelming and may lead to feelings of uncertainty and fear. However, finding meaning and purpose can be a powerful tool in navigating the challenges of living with pancreatic cancer.

Embracing the Present Moment

One way to find meaning and purpose is by embracing the present moment. Pancreatic cancer can make us acutely aware of the fragility of life and the importance of cherishing each day. By focusing on the present, we can find joy in the simple things and appreciate the beauty that surrounds us.

Take a moment each day to practice mindfulness. This involves bringing your attention to the present moment without judgment. Whether it's through meditation, deep breathing exercises, or simply taking a walk in nature, mindfulness can help you cultivate a sense of gratitude and find meaning in the here and now.

Reflecting on Personal Values

Another way to find meaning and purpose is by reflecting on your personal values. What is truly important to you? What gives your life meaning? Take some time to explore these questions and identify the values that resonate with you.

Once you have identified your values, strive to align your actions with them. For example, if family is important to you, make an effort to spend quality time with your loved ones. If creativity brings you joy, engage in activities that allow you to express your artistic side. By living in accordance with your values, you can find a sense of purpose and fulfillment, even in the face of pancreatic cancer.

Engaging in Meaningful Activities

Engaging in meaningful activities can also provide a sense of purpose and fulfillment. These activities can vary greatly from person to person, so it's important to find what resonates with you. It could be volunteering for a cause you care about, pursuing a hobby or passion, or even starting a new project or venture.

Finding meaning and purpose doesn't mean you have to take on grand endeavors. Sometimes, the smallest acts of kindness or moments of connection can have a profound impact. Look for opportunities to make a difference in the lives of others, whether it's through a kind word, a helping hand, or a listening ear. These acts of compassion can bring a sense of purpose and meaning to your own life.

Seeking Support and Connection

Finding meaning and purpose is not a journey you have to embark on alone. Seek support from your loved ones, friends, or even support groups specifically for individuals living with pancreatic cancer. Connecting with others who are going through similar experiences can provide a sense of belonging and understanding.

Consider joining a support group where you can share your thoughts, fears, and triumphs with others who truly understand. These connections can offer valuable insights, encouragement, and a sense of community. Together, you can explore ways to find meaning and purpose in your lives, even in the face of pancreatic cancer.

Embracing the Power of Hope

Hope is a powerful force that can help us find meaning and purpose amid adversity. It is important to cultivate hope and hold onto it, even when faced with the challenges of pancreatic cancer. Hope can motivate you to keep moving forward, to seek out new treatments, and to embrace life to the fullest.

Find sources of inspiration that resonate with you. It could be reading books, listening to uplifting music, or watching movies that touch your heart. Surround yourself with positive influences that remind you of the beauty and resilience of the human spirit.

Embracing the Journey

Living with pancreatic cancer is undoubtedly a challenging journey, but it can also be an opportunity for growth, self-discovery, and finding meaning and purpose. Embrace the journey and allow yourself to explore new perspectives, beliefs, and experiences.

Remember, finding meaning and purpose is a deeply personal process. What brings meaning to one person may be different for another. Take the time to reflect, explore, and listen to your inner voice. Trust that you have the strength and resilience to navigate this journey and find meaning and purpose along the way.

In the next section, we will explore strategies for dealing with anxiety and depression, which are common emotional challenges faced by individuals living with pancreatic cancer.

Dealing with Anxiety and Depression

Receiving a diagnosis of pancreatic cancer can be overwhelming and can bring about a range of emotions, including anxiety and depression. It is completely normal to experience these feelings, as a cancer diagnosis can be a life-altering event. However, it is important to remember that you are not alone in this journey, and there are strategies and support available to help you navigate through these challenging emotions.

Understanding Anxiety and Depression

Anxiety and depression are common emotional responses to a cancer diagnosis. Anxiety is characterized by feelings of worry, fear, and unease, often accompanied by physical symptoms such as restlessness, difficulty concentrating, and trouble sleeping. Depression, on the other hand, involves persistent feelings of sadness, hopelessness, and a loss of interest in once-enjoyable activities.

It is important to recognize that anxiety and depression can have a significant impact on your overall well-being and quality of life. They can affect your ability to cope with treatment, make decisions, and maintain relationships. Therefore, it is crucial to address these emotions and seek support.

Seeking Support

Dealing with anxiety and depression on your own can be challenging. It is important to reach out to your healthcare team, friends, and family for support. They can provide a listening ear, offer encouragement, and help you navigate through the emotional challenges that come with a cancer diagnosis.

In addition to your loved ones, consider joining a support group specifically for individuals with pancreatic cancer. These groups provide a safe space to share experiences, learn coping strategies from others who have been through similar situations, and gain a sense of community. Support groups can be in-person or online, depending on your preference and availability.

Therapy and Counseling

Therapy and counseling can be valuable tools for managing anxiety and depression. A therapist or counselor can help you explore and understand your emotions, develop coping mechanisms, and guide you on how to navigate through the challenges of living with pancreatic cancer.

Cognitive-behavioral therapy (CBT) is a common approach used to address anxiety and depression. CBT focuses on identifying and changing negative thought patterns and behaviors that contribute to these emotions. By challenging and reframing negative thoughts, you can develop a more positive and resilient mindset.

Relaxation Techniques

Incorporating relaxation techniques into your daily routine can help alleviate anxiety and depression. Deep breathing exercises, meditation, and progressive muscle relaxation are effective techniques that can promote a sense of calm and reduce stress.

Deep breathing exercises involve taking slow, deep breaths and focusing on the sensation of the breath entering and leaving your body. This simple practice can help slow down your heart rate and relax your mind.

Meditation involves focusing your attention and eliminating the stream of thoughts that may be causing anxiety or depression. There are various forms of meditation, such as mindfulness meditation, guided imagery, and loving-kindness meditation. Find a technique that resonates with you and practice it regularly to experience its benefits.

Progressive muscle relaxation involves tensing and then releasing different muscle groups in your body. This technique helps you become more aware of tension and teaches you how to relax your muscles, promoting a sense of physical and mental relaxation.

Engaging in Activities You Enjoy

Engaging in activities that bring you joy and fulfillment can help combat anxiety and depression. Whether it's pursuing a hobby, spending time in nature, listening to music, or practicing art, finding activities that uplift your spirits can provide a much-needed distraction from the challenges of living with pancreatic cancer.

It is important to remember that self-care is not selfish. Taking time for yourself and engaging in activities that bring you happiness can have a positive impact on your mental well-being.

Medication

In some cases, medication may be prescribed to help manage anxiety and depression. Antidepressant medications can help regulate brain chemicals that affect mood and emotions. It is important to discuss the potential benefits and side effects of medication with your healthcare team to determine if it is the right option for you.

Building a Supportive Network

Building a supportive network of friends, family, and healthcare professionals is crucial to managing anxiety and depression. Surrounding yourself with positive and understanding individuals who can provide emotional support can make a significant difference in your well-being.

Additionally, consider reaching out to organizations and resources that specialize in providing support for individuals with pancreatic cancer. These organizations often offer counseling services, educational materials, and online communities where you can connect with others who are going through similar experiences.

Dealing with anxiety and depression while living with pancreatic cancer can be challenging, but it is important to remember that you are not alone. Seeking support, whether it's from loved ones, therapy, relaxation techniques, engaging in activities you enjoy, or medication, can help you navigate through these emotions and improve your overall well-being. Remember to be kind to yourself and prioritize self-care as you continue on your journey of thriving with pancreatic cancer.

Chapter 5

Living a Fulfilling Life with Pancreatic Cancer

Setting Goals and Priorities

When faced with a diagnosis of pancreatic cancer, it is natural to feel overwhelmed and uncertain about the future. However, setting goals and priorities can provide a sense of direction and purpose, helping you navigate through the challenges ahead. In this section, we will explore the importance of setting goals, how to identify your priorities, and strategies for achieving them.

The Power of Setting Goals

Setting goals is a powerful tool that can help you regain a sense of control and focus during your pancreatic cancer journey. Goals provide a roadmap for your actions and decisions, giving you something to strive for and look forward to. They can also serve as a source of motivation and inspiration, reminding you of what is truly important to you.

When setting goals, it is essential to keep in mind that they should be realistic and achievable. While it is important to aim high, setting unrealistic goals can lead to frustration and disappointment. Instead, break your goals down into smaller, manageable steps that you can work towards. This will not only make them more attainable but also allow you to celebrate your progress along the way.

Identifying Your Priorities

To set meaningful goals, it is crucial to identify your priorities. Take some time to reflect on what matters most to you in your life. Consider your values, passions, and the things that bring you joy and fulfillment. This process can help you gain clarity and guide your decision-making as you navigate through your pancreatic cancer journey.

It is also important to recognize that your priorities may shift as you go through different stages of your treatment and recovery. What may have been a priority before your diagnosis may no longer hold the same significance. Be open to reassessing and adjusting your priorities as needed, allowing yourself the flexibility to adapt to changing circumstances.

Strategies for Achieving Your Goals

Once you have identified your goals and priorities, it is time to develop strategies for achieving them. Here are some strategies that can help you stay focused and make progress toward your goals:

1. **Break it down:** Break your goals down into smaller, manageable tasks. This will make them less overwhelming and more achievable. Create a timeline or action plan to guide your progress.

2. **Seek support:** Don't be afraid to ask for help and lean on your support network. Friends, family, and healthcare professionals can provide valuable guidance, encouragement, and assistance along the way.

3. **Celebrate milestones:** Celebrate your achievements, no matter how small they may seem. Recognize and reward yourself for the progress you have made. This will help boost your motivation and keep you inspired.

4. **Stay positive:** Maintain a positive mindset and focus on the possibilities rather than the limitations. Surround yourself with positivity, and seek out sources of inspiration and encouragement.

5. **Practice self-care:** Taking care of yourself is essential when working towards your goals. Prioritize self-care activities such as exercise, relaxation techniques, and engaging in hobbies that bring you joy and peace.

6. **Stay flexible:** Be open to adjusting your goals and strategies as needed. Life is unpredictable, and circumstances may change. Embrace flexibility and adaptability to ensure your goals remain relevant and achievable.

Remember, setting goals is not about adding more pressure or stress to your life. It is about creating a sense of purpose and direction, helping you live a fulfilling life despite the challenges of pancreatic cancer. By setting goals and identifying your priorities, you can take an active role in shaping your journey and finding meaning and joy along the way.

Maintaining Relationships and Intimacy

When facing a diagnosis of pancreatic cancer, it's natural to focus on your well-being and treatment. However, it's important to remember that maintaining relationships and intimacy with your loved ones can play a significant role in your overall well-being and quality of life. Cancer can put a strain on relationships, but with open communication, understanding, and support, you can navigate this challenging journey together.

The Impact of Pancreatic Cancer on Relationships

A diagnosis of pancreatic cancer can have a profound impact on your relationships with family, friends, and even your partner. It's common for both you and your loved ones to experience a range of emotions, including fear, sadness, anger, and uncertainty. These emotions can sometimes lead to tension and strain in your relationships.

It's important to remember that everyone copes with difficult situations differently. Your loved ones may have their own fears and concerns about your diagnosis, and they may struggle to find the right words or actions to support you. Likewise, you may find it challenging to express your own emotions and needs while dealing with the physical and emotional toll of cancer.

Open and Honest Communication

One of the most crucial aspects of maintaining relationships during this time is open and honest communication. It's essential to express your feelings, fears and needs to your loved ones and to listen to their concerns as well. By sharing your thoughts and emotions, you can create a safe space for open dialogue and understanding.

It's important to remember that your loved ones may not always know how to support you, and they may need guidance from you. Be clear about what you need, whether it's a listening ear, practical help, or simply someone to accompany you to medical appointments. By communicating your needs, you can strengthen your relationships and ensure that your loved ones feel involved and valued in your journey.

Nurturing Intimacy

Intimacy is an essential part of any relationship, and it can be challenging to maintain when facing a diagnosis of pancreatic cancer. Physical and emotional changes, as well as the stress of treatment, can impact your desire for intimacy. However, it's important to remember that intimacy is not solely about physical intimacy but also about emotional connection and closeness.

Communication plays a vital role in nurturing intimacy. Talk openly with your partner about your concerns, fears, and desires. Discuss any physical changes or limitations you may be experiencing, and explore alternative ways to express affection and closeness. Remember that intimacy can take many forms, such as holding hands, cuddling, or simply spending quality time together.

Seeking Support

Maintaining relationships and intimacy can be challenging, and it's essential to seek support when needed. Consider joining a support group for cancer patients and their loved ones. These groups provide a safe space to share experiences, gain insights, and receive emotional support from others who understand what you're going through.

Individual counseling or couples therapy can also be beneficial in navigating the challenges that arise from a pancreatic cancer diagnosis. A trained therapist can help you and your loved ones communicate effectively, manage emotions, and find strategies to maintain intimacy and connection.

Balancing Self-care and Relationships

While it's important to maintain relationships and intimacy, it's equally crucial to prioritize self-care. Taking care of your physical and emotional well-being is essential for your overall health and ability to support your loved ones.

Set boundaries and communicate your needs for alone time or rest. It's okay to ask for help and delegate tasks to your loved ones when necessary. Remember that taking care of yourself allows you to be present and engaged in your relationships.

Embracing Moments of Joy

Amidst the challenges of pancreatic cancer, it's important to embrace moments of joy and create positive memories with your loved ones. Plan activities or outings that bring you happiness and allow you to connect with your loved ones on a deeper level. Whether it's a family gathering, a picnic in the park, or a movie night at home, these moments can provide a much-needed respite from the difficulties of cancer.

Exploring Palliative Care and Hospice

When facing a diagnosis of pancreatic cancer, it's important to consider all aspects of your care, including palliative care and hospice. These two forms of care are often misunderstood and can be associated with end-of-life care. However, they offer much more than that and can greatly enhance your quality of life throughout your cancer journey.

Understanding Palliative Care

Palliative care focuses on providing relief from the symptoms and side effects of pancreatic cancer, as well as addressing the emotional and psychological challenges that come with the disease. It is a specialized form of medical care that aims to improve your overall well-being and help you maintain the best possible quality of life.

Palliative care can be provided at any stage of your cancer journey, from the time of diagnosis through treatment and beyond. It is not limited to end-of-life care and can be integrated with curative treatments. The goal is to manage pain, control symptoms, and improve your overall comfort and quality of life.

A palliative care team typically consists of healthcare professionals such as doctors, nurses, social workers, and psychologists who work together to provide comprehensive support. They will collaborate with your primary oncology team to ensure that your physical, emotional, and spiritual needs are met.

The Benefits of Palliative Care

Engaging in palliative care can bring numerous benefits to pancreatic cancer patients. Here are some key advantages:

1. Symptom Management

Pancreatic cancer and its treatments can cause a range of symptoms, including pain, nausea, fatigue, and loss of appetite. Palliative care specialists are skilled in managing these symptoms and can work with you to develop a personalized plan to alleviate your discomfort. By effectively managing your symptoms, you can experience a better quality of life and maintain your ability to engage in daily activities.

2. Emotional and Psychological Support

A pancreatic cancer diagnosis can be emotionally overwhelming, and it's crucial to have support in navigating the complex emotions that arise. Palliative care teams include psychologists and social workers who can provide counseling and emotional support to help you cope with the challenges you face. They can also assist in addressing any anxiety, depression, or other mental health concerns that may arise during your cancer journey.

3. Communication and Decision-Making

Palliative care teams are skilled at facilitating open and honest communication between patients, families, and healthcare providers. They can help you understand your treatment options, discuss your goals and priorities, and assist in making informed decisions about your care. By having these conversations, you can ensure that your treatment aligns with your values and preferences.

4. Coordination of Care

Managing pancreatic cancer often involves multiple healthcare providers and treatments. Palliative care teams can help coordinate your care, ensuring that all aspects of your treatment plan are integrated and well-managed. They can also assist in coordinating appointments, medications, and other supportive services, reducing the burden on you and your loved ones.

Understanding Hospice Care

Hospice care is a specialized form of care that focuses on providing comfort and support to individuals with a life-limiting illness, including pancreatic cancer. It is typically offered when curative treatments are no longer effective or desired, and the focus shifts to maximizing quality of life in the final stages of the disease.

Hospice care can be provided in various settings, including your own home, a hospice facility, or a hospital. The primary goal is to ensure that you are comfortable and free from pain, while also addressing your emotional and spiritual needs. Hospice care is provided by a team of healthcare professionals who specialize in end-of-life care.

The Benefits of Hospice Care

While hospice care is often associated with the end of life, it offers numerous benefits for both patients and their families:

1. Comfort and Pain Management

Hospice care focuses on providing comfort and relieving pain. The team of healthcare professionals will work closely with you to manage your symptoms and ensure that you are as comfortable as possible. This can greatly enhance your quality of life during the final stages of pancreatic cancer.

2. Emotional and Spiritual Support

Hospice care recognizes the importance of addressing emotional and spiritual needs during the end-of-life journey. The team will provide emotional support to both you and your loved ones, helping you navigate the complex emotions that arise during this time. They can also assist in connecting you with spiritual resources, if desired.

3. Assistance for Caregivers

Hospice care extends support not only to patients but also to their caregivers. The team can provide education, respite care, and emotional support to help caregivers navigate the challenges of providing care and coping with their own emotions. This can alleviate some of the burden and stress associated with caregiving.

4. Bereavement Support

After the passing of a loved one, hospice care continues to offer support to the family. Bereavement services are provided to help loved ones cope with grief and loss. This can include counseling, support groups, and resources to assist in the healing process.

Making Informed Decisions

When considering palliative care and hospice, it's important to have open and honest conversations with your healthcare team and loved ones. Discuss your goals, concerns, and preferences to ensure that the care you receive aligns with your values and wishes.

Remember, palliative care can be integrated with curative treatments, and hospice care is not limited to the final days or weeks of life. Both forms of care can greatly enhance your quality of life and provide the support you need throughout your pancreatic cancer journey.

By exploring palliative care and hospice, you can ensure that you are receiving comprehensive care that addresses all aspects of your well-being. Embracing these forms of care can help you thrive and find comfort and support during this challenging time.

Finding Hope and Inspiration

Receiving a diagnosis of pancreatic cancer can be overwhelming and can leave you feeling scared and uncertain about the future. It's completely normal to experience a range of emotions during this time. However, it's important to remember that there is always hope and inspiration to be found, even in the face of such a challenging diagnosis.

Embracing Positivity

Maintaining a positive mindset can make a significant difference in your overall well-being and quality of life. While it may be difficult at times, finding hope and inspiration can help you navigate through the ups and downs of your pancreatic cancer journey.

One way to embrace positivity is by surrounding yourself with supportive and uplifting people. Seek out friends, family members, or support groups that can provide encouragement and understanding. Sharing your experiences and hearing the stories of others who have overcome similar challenges can be incredibly empowering.

Seeking Inspiration from Others

Finding inspiration from others who have faced pancreatic cancer can be a powerful source of hope. There are numerous stories of individuals who have not only survived but thrived despite their diagnosis. These stories can serve as a reminder that you are not alone and that there is always a possibility for a positive outcome.

Consider reading books, articles, or blogs written by pancreatic cancer survivors. Their experiences and insights can provide valuable guidance and inspiration. Additionally, attending support groups or connecting with online communities can introduce you to individuals who have successfully navigated their pancreatic cancer journey.

Exploring Alternative Therapies

In addition to conventional medical treatments, many individuals with pancreatic cancer explore alternative therapies to complement their treatment plans. While it's important to consult with your healthcare team before trying any alternative therapies, some individuals find hope and inspiration in these approaches.

Alternative therapies such as acupuncture, massage, meditation, and yoga have been reported to provide physical and emotional benefits for cancer patients. These practices can help reduce stress, improve sleep, and enhance overall well-being. Exploring these therapies may not only provide relief from symptoms but also offer a sense of hope and control over your healing process.

Engaging in Creative Outlets

Engaging in creative outlets can be a powerful way to find hope and inspiration during your pancreatic cancer journey. Whether it's painting, writing, playing music, or any other form of artistic expression, these activities can provide a sense of purpose and joy.

Creativity allows you to focus on something other than your diagnosis and treatment, giving you a much-needed break from the challenges you may be facing. It can also serve as a form of therapy, allowing you to express your emotions and find solace in the process.

Connecting with Nature

Nature has a remarkable ability to inspire and uplift the human spirit. Spending time outdoors, whether it's taking a walk in a park, sitting by the beach, or simply enjoying the beauty of a garden, can have a profound impact on your well-being.

Nature provides a sense of peace and tranquility, allowing you to momentarily escape from the stress and worries of your diagnosis. It can also remind you of the beauty and resilience of life, offering hope and inspiration during difficult times.

Finding Meaning and Purpose

Finding meaning and purpose in your life can be a powerful source of hope and inspiration. Take the time to reflect on what truly matters to you and what brings you joy and fulfillment. This may involve reevaluating your priorities, setting new goals, or pursuing activities that align with your values.

Engaging in acts of kindness and giving back to others can also provide a sense of purpose. Whether it's volunteering, supporting a cause you believe in, or simply offering a listening ear to someone in need, these acts can bring a deep sense of fulfillment and inspire hope in both yourself and others.

Cultivating Inner Strength

Pancreatic cancer may test your physical and emotional strength, but it can also help you discover a reservoir of inner strength you never knew you had. Cultivating this inner strength involves developing resilience, practicing self-compassion, and embracing the power of your mind.

Resilience allows you to bounce back from setbacks and challenges, while self-compassion reminds you to be kind and gentle with yourself during difficult times. Embracing the power of your mind involves harnessing the strength of positive thinking, visualization, and affirmations to create a mindset that supports your healing journey.

Embracing the Present Moment

Lastly, finding hope and inspiration often involves embracing the present moment. While it's natural to worry about the future, focusing on the present can help you appreciate the small joys and blessings in your life.

Take the time to savor simple pleasures, such as spending time with loved ones, enjoying a delicious meal, or witnessing a beautiful sunset. By immersing yourself in the present moment, you can find hope and inspiration in the beauty and wonder that surrounds you.

Remember, finding hope and inspiration is a personal journey, and what works for one person may not work for another. Explore different strategies, listen to your intuition, and trust that you have the strength and resilience to navigate through your pancreatic cancer journey with hope and inspiration.

Conclusion

The pancreatic cancer journey, while intensely difficult, can be an opportunity to embrace life and health in new ways. As Sam's story illustrates, there are many ways to thrive physically and emotionally while navigating this diagnosis.

This book has provided evidence-based strategies to support you or your loved one through every stage, from understanding the disease to fostering well-being during treatment to transitioning into life as a survivor. While the cancer itself cannot be controlled, you have the power to impact your healing path.

The integrative approaches covered, including anticancer nutrition, stress management, physical activity, and mindset shifts, can help patients defy the odds. By viewing this as a catalyst to implement positive lifestyle changes and refocus priorities, it is possible to find meaning in the cancer experience.

While the reality of pancreatic cancer is challenging, real hope comes from the human capacity to grow through adversity. You have the inner strength needed to not only survive but thrive in body, mind, and spirit. Focus on the factors within your control and take this journey one step at a time, armed with information and support.

You are greater than this diagnosis. Allow the strategies in this book to point you towards healing, empowerment, and living life abundantly. Stay connected to resources, maintain perspective, celebrate each victory, and know you have the resilience to meet this challenge. Thriving with pancreatic cancer starts now, with active partnership, courage, and hope.